*Your Colon—Learn about
It for a Better Life*

YOUR COLON— LEARN ABOUT IT FOR A BETTER LIFE

John E. Cogan, M.D.

VANTAGE PRESS
New York / Los Angeles / Chicago

Published by Vantage Press, Inc.
516 West 34th Street, New York, New York 10001

Manufactured in the United States of America
ISBN: 0-533-07817-2

Library of Congress Catalog Card No.: 87-90275

To my beloved wife, Naomi,
and my daughters,
Robin and Laura

Contents

Preface

I am a doctor who has been practicing colon and rectal surgery and diagnosis of diseases of the colon and rectum for the past twenty-four years. I have written this book to inform laypeople on certain aspects of the colon, so that with this knowledge they can understand their bodily functions better and possibly help their regularity as far as bowel habits are concerned. Over the past twenty-four years, I have been asked a lot of questions concerning the colon and its function, and I have given a lot of answers to these questions. Of the thousands of questions that I have written down that people have asked me, I have picked out the more consistent questions and have entered them into this book in a format that should be easy to read. A person may turn to any page or chapter in this book and may possibly find the questions and answers on any subject concerning the colon and rectum. I have tried to make the answer concise yet complete. It is interesting to note, in talking to thousands of patients over the years, their misconceptions of very popular maladies such as hemorrhoids, fissures, and cancer. I am hoping that this easy-reading book, with its questions and answers, will enlighten the public on this very important subject of the colon and the rectum. Whereas some people will think about their colon only two or three minutes a day, other people will agonize over their colon and rectum for hours each day, allowing the colon to run their lives rather than for the person to control their colon. I feel that the knowledge imparted in this book should help a lot of people have a happier and healthier life.

*Your Colon—Learn about
It for a Better Life*

Chapter I

Anatomy
(What Are Your Colon and Rectum?)

QUESTION: What are my colon and rectum?

ANSWER: The intestinal tract, starting with your mouth and going to your anal opening, is approximately thirty feet in length. The last five feet of this intestinal organ is called the colon, and the last seven to eight inches of the colon is called the rectum, and the last two inches of the colon is called the anal canal.

QUESTION: Where are the colon and rectum in the abdominal cavity?

ANSWER: The colon begins on the lower right side of your abdominal cavity, located approximately where your appendix would be. It then travels upward to under your right rib cage; then it traverses across the upper abdomen to the area of your abdominal cavity, under your left ribs. The colon then proceeds downward to your left hip area and then goes over to the middle of the abdominal cavity, to approximately the middle of your bladder. The colon then proceeds to go out through the pelvis as your rectum and anus. The colon is situated in your abdominal cavity like an inverted horseshoe.

1

QUESTION: Since some people call the colon the lower intestine, does that mean it sits low in the abdominal cavity?

ANSWER: No. Because this organ is also called the lower intestine, this does not mean it sits low in the abdominal cavity. As described above, the colon can be as high up as the lower limits of your rib cage. This myth is perpetuated because the colon is the last five feet of the intestinal tract and thus is incorrectly thought to be low in the abdominal cavity.

QUESTION: Are there various names for parts of the colon?

ANSWER: Yes, the colon has names designating which portion one is speaking about. The portion of the colon that starts over on the right side, where the appendix is attached to the colon, is called the cecum. The cecum then enters into the ascending colon or right colon, which comes up under the right rib cage. As it turns to go across the body, this turn is called the hepatic flexure, for it is adjacent to the liver. The portion that swings across the upper abdomen to the left side is called the transverse colon. As it makes a turn to go down to the left pelvis, this portion is called the splenic flexure because it is adjacent to the spleen. As the colon then traverses down the left side of the body, it is called the descending colon, and then that portion of the colon that goes from the left lower quadrant of the abdomen to the lower middle of the body is called the sigmoid colon. The segment of the sigmoid colon then in the middle of the lower body goes into the rectum, which comes out of the abdominal cavity as the rectum and, last but not least, the anal canal.

QUESTION: Can a person live without a colon and rectum?

ANSWER: Yes, the body can function perfectly normally without the colon and rectum; however, the person will have a slight handicap called an ileostomy, which is a small piece of small intestine that protrudes through the abdominal wall, and the patient has to wear a bag around the intestinal opening (ileostomy) in order to catch the waste material.

QUESTION: What is the function of the colon?

ANSWER: The colon has several functions; however, the two most important functions are: (1) to absorb the water out of the waste material, so that a person passes a solid stool, and (2) to store the stool in the left portion of the colon, ready for evacuation.

QUESTION: If water is drawn out of the waste material by the colon, where does the fluid go?

ANSWER: When the colon absorbs the fluid out of the waste material, it provides the cells of the body with this fluid, especially if a person has not had enough fluid intake.

QUESTION: I have given myself a regular tap water enema and have held it for thirty minutes and have never been able to pass the water out. Is this possible?

ANSWER: Yes, if you tend to be on the dehydrated side, the colon will absorb the quart of water into the cells of your body, and you will not have any fluid to evacuate.

QUESTION: Because a portion of the colon is up under my ribs, is it true that a person can have a gas pain or spasm in this portion of colon and it can simulate a heart attack or gallbladder attack?

ANSWER: Yes, a person may have a spasm or an accumulation of gas in the transverse colon, and the pain can simulate a heart attack or a gallbladder attack.

QUESTION: What does the term *redundant colon* mean in an otherwise negative colon X ray?

ANSWER: A redundant colon means that you have some extra colon that you were born with, and this has little adverse reaction on the function of the colon; it is a variation of the norm. It is like having big feet or a large nose, which is merely a variation in body organs.

QUESTION: Does the colon have bacteria in it?

ANSWER: Yes, the colon has bacteria in it, which helps with the fermentation of the waste material. As long as the bacteria remain in the colon, they are very helpful; however, should the bacteria in the colon in some way, by trauma or disease, get access to the abdominal cavity, then this can set up a very serious disease called peritonitis.

QUESTION: Now and then I will hear the word *borborygmi* mentioned in connection with the colon. What is this?

ANSWER: Borborygmi are the sounds that are made by the contraction of the colon.

QUESTION: What makes the funny noises that I can hear in my intestinal tract?

ANSWER: These funny noises are contractions of the small or large intestinal tract and are usually caused either by certain foods or liquids that we ingest or can be brought about by stress and worry in our lives.

QUESTION: Is there any difference between the female colon and the male colon?

ANSWER: Yes, the female colon is usually larger than the male colon, and this is the reason that most females have different bowel habits than the typical male.

QUESTION: Does this different size in the male and the female colon have a direct correlation to the type and frequency of male and female bowel movements?

ANSWER: Since the female colon is larger, it can hold more stool and for a longer time. The typical normal female bowel movement is every two or three days, is larger than the male stool, and is dryer than the male stool. The female usually strains at the beginning of her bowel movement to start the bowel movement and is still straining to evacuate all of her bowel movement that day. The male colon, being small, cannot store as much stool or absorb as much water; therefore, the typical normal male has a bowel movement every day and sometimes twice a day. It is usually firm at first and then semisolid, and the male usually has a much easier bowel movement each day than does the female.

QUESTION: Do the colon and rectum have any feeling?

ANSWER: The only feeling the colon and rectum have is distention; otherwise, the outer layer and inner layer of the colon and intestinal tract have no feeling to them at all. If a person swallows a nail or an open safety pin and these objects perforate the colon, there will be no feeling until infection sets in. A doctor in his office may cauterize the lining of the bowel, and there will be no feeling of the hot cautery touching the lining of the colon. The growth up in the colon may be completely removed through the colonoscopy instrument, and there will be absolutely no feeling except for the discomfort of the tube in the rectum.

QUESTION: When having a normal bowel movement, does a person empty out his entire colon of waste material?

ANSWER: No. When a person has a bowel movement, only approximately eight to ten inches of stool is evacuated from the rectum, and the remainder of the waste material remains in the colon.

QUESTION: How does blood supply get to the colon?

ANSWER: There is some fatty tissue formed like an apron that comes off of one side of the colon, which is called the "mesentery." It is attached to one side of the colon and to the back of the abdominal cavity. This mesentery contains the arteries and veins that supply the colon with its blood.

QUESTION: Are there lymph nodes in the area of the colon?

ANSWER: Yes, there are lymph nodes in the area of the colon that drain the colon and are situated in the mesentery of the colon. They belong to a separate circulatory system called the "lymphatic sytem," and this system contains nodes. This system is very important in determining the spread of cancer of the colon and rectum.

QUESTION: What is the composition of the wall of the colon?

ANSWER: The wall of the colon is made up of an inner layer called the "mucosa," which is lined with glandular cells that have the ability to absorb water. The middle layer is made up of muscular tissue, and the outer layer is called the "serosa," which is the outer cover of the colon. These layers are important because certain tumors can arise from each of these layers, and each tumor has different characteristics that dictate how fast they grow, how they spread, and how they should be treated.

QUESTION: Are there other names for the colon?

ANSWER: Yes, the colon is also called the large bowel or large intestine or lower bowel.

QUESTION: Why does the colon look like a link sausage?

ANSWER: Because the colon is divided up into short segments called "haustral segments" that contract and expand and move the stool along the colon.

QUESTION: When waste material empties from the small intestine into the large intestine, how long does it take the waste material to travel the five feet of large intestine or colon?

ANSWER: The average time that the waste material takes from the cecum or right side of the colon to the rectum is approximately twenty-four to forty-eight hours. Some food products take longer or shorter, but the myth that the food you eat today you evacuate tomorrow is generally wrong.

QUESTION: Food goes through the small intestine in twenty-five minutes and empties into the colon as a liquid. Does it stay a liquid?

ANSWER: The waste material when it reaches the colon is in a liquid form and becomes a solid as it travels around the five feet of colon.

Chapter II

Itching and Irritation

QUESTION: As a proctologist (colon and rectal specialist), what is the most common ailment that you have seen in your practice in the past twenty-four years?

ANSWER: Itching and irritation around the anal and perianal area are the most common complaints that I hear in my office year after year.

QUESTION: What is the most common cause of itching and irritation in the anal and perianal area?

ANSWER: In my practice over the past twenty-four years, 99 percent of all itching and irritation was caused by diet. The other 1 percent is usually caused by many factors, such as oral antibiotics, applying soap to the area, perfumed or colored toilet tissue; or organic pathology, such as hemorrhoids, fissures, and fistulas.

QUESTION: Does this mean that hemorrhoids rarely cause itching and irritation?

ANSWER: Correct. In 99 percent of cases of hemorrhoids, we could remove the hemorrhoids and the patient would still have the itching and irritation. In my practice the so-called itching hemorrhoids are very rare.

QUESTION: Does this mean that a person should not have his hemorrhoids removed for the symptom of itching alone?

ANSWER: Correct. Removal of the hemorrhoids rarely cures the itching.

QUESTION: If 99 percent of all itching and irritation around the anal area is caused by diet, does this mean that the patient is allergic to certain food products?

ANSWER: Yes, the person can be allergic to certain food products, some if ingested on only one occasion, but usually requiring eating the food product three or four days in a row.

QUESTION: What are some of the common food products from which people will get irritation and itching in the anal area?

ANSWER: The following food products will generally cause itching and irritation if ingested consecutively for several days: nuts, pork, chocolate, alcohol, highly seasoned foods, shell seafoods, fresh fruit, and milk.

QUESTION: I thought fresh fruit was a good, healthy food for a person.

ANSWER: In general, fresh fruit is healthy for the body. Fresh fruit in some people, if eaten consecutively for several days, will cause an anal itching and irritation.

QUESTION: Can itching and irritation be a year-round problem for a patient?

ANSWER: Yes, I find that in the springtime patients who raise their own fresh fruit in a garden will have a lot of anal itching and irritation. Patients who eat a lot of fresh fruit, such as cantaloupe and watermelon in the summertime, will have a lot of problems. Deer hunters in the fall who go out to hunt venison and make venison sausage, which is half pork, will have a lot of irritation. At Christmastime people will eat a lot of rich foods, perhaps including a box of grapefruit from the Texas Valley, which will give them anal and perianal itching and irritation in the month of January.

QUESTION: Will a cream or ointment alone resolve the problem of itching or irritation in a patient?

ANSWER: No, giving a patient a cream or an ointment to apply to the area will bring only temporary relief. The cause of the problem must be diagnosed. If it is a food product, then this food product must be identified. The patient is then given a set of instructions to follow and medications to use and is instructed to omit the harmful food product for three weeks, until the itching and irritation are resolved. The patient may then eat the suspicious food product in moderation.

QUESTION: What are some helpful rules to obey in order to avoid anal and perianal itching and irritation?

ANSWER: One of the best home remedies for itching and irritation is to cleanse the area with the over-the-counter product witch hazel several times a day. Other helpful hints are to avoid diarrhea and not to apply any type of soap directly to the anal or perianal area at any time. It is also helpful to keep the area dry by applying baby powder or cornstarch daily. A good over-the-counter hydrocortisone cream or one prescribed by your doctor will help this problem greatly. Always use a cream and not an ointment on the area because a cream will dry out and ointment will not. One of the main objects of the treatment is to keep the area dry.

QUESTION: Can you name something subtle that may cause irritation around the anal area?

ANSWER: Yes. Once I had a patient who increased her vitamin C (ascorbic acid) during the wintertime, hoping not to get the flu, and she developed an intolerable rash around the anal and perianal area from the increased intake of vitamin C.

QUESTION: Is it beneficial to use a topical anesthetic to relieve the itching and irritation, if only temporarily?

ANSWER: It is very common for people to be allergic to the "caine" derivative in topical anesthetics; thus, they will only compound their problem by using a topical anesthetic.

QUESTION: Why do people scratch an itch?

ANSWER: Because a person generally cannot tolerate itching; however, if by scratching he can turn the itch into pain, then the pain is more tolerable.

QUESTION: Do people usually overtreat itching and irritation in the anal area?

ANSWER: Yes. Itching can become so intolerable in that area that people tend to overtreat and scratch, and by the time I see them it looks as if they had used a steel brush in the area.

QUESTION: How bad can the itching and irritation get?

ANSWER: One patient said if I couldn't help him clear up the itching, would I please give him eight more hands to scratch with.

Chapter III

Hemorrhoids

QUESTION: What are hemorrhoids?

ANSWER: Hemorrhoids are varicose veins, both inside the anal canal and outside the anal canal.

QUESTION: What percentage of patients whom you see in your practice have hemorrhoids?

ANSWER: Approximately two-thirds of all the patients I see will have some degree of hemorrhoids, either internal or external.

QUESTION: What causes hemorrhoids?

ANSWER: Hemorrhoids are almost 100 percent an inherited trait. Keep in mind while reading these answers that there is a big difference between the words *cause* and *aggravate.*

QUESTION: Do more men or more women have hemorrhoids?

ANSWER: More men have hemorrhoids.

QUESTION: I thought pregnancy caused hemorrhoids.

ANSWER: No. Pregnancy will aggravate hemorrhoids in a female who already has them, but it does not cause hemorrhoids.

QUESTION: Why do so many women insist that either when carrying their baby or at time of delivery they develop hemorrhoids?

ANSWER: This is because females who are pregnant and have hemorrhoids many times will develop a complication of those hemorrhoids, which can be quite painful, and it is these complications that give the patient the impression that the pregnancy caused the hemorrhoids.

QUESTION: What is the most common complication of hemorrhoids during pregnancy?

ANSWER: A thrombotic hemorrhoid, or the development of a blood clot in a hemorrhoidal vein.

QUESTION: Can this complication occur without being pregnant?

ANSWER: Yes. Thrombotic hemorrhoids are very common in men and women of all ages.

QUESTION: Exactly what is a thrombotic hemorrhoid and what should a person expect from it if not treated?

ANSWER: A thrombotic hemorrhoid may present itself very rapidly as a painful swelling around the anal opening. From day one, when it appears, the pain will generally last from three to five days, becoming less severe each day. The swelling or blood clot itself will slowly be absorbed by the body, and it will take generally two or three weeks for the knot to disappear; however, the patient still has the hemorrhoids; the complication has merely resolved itself.

QUESTION: Do thrombotic hemorrhoids bleed?

ANSWER: If the patient develops a thrombotic hemorrhoid and continues to be active, including sports, there is a chance that because of the rubbing of the buttocks together a small hole may develop in the thrombotic hemorrhoid and the clot will slowly ooze out over a few days' time.

QUESTION: Does this mean that thrombotic hemorrhoids, starting from the minute they appear, will begin to resolve themselves regardless of treatment?

ANSWER: Yes. Small blood clots not too painful can usually be treated symptomatically with over-the-counter medications. Larger, more painful clots should be treated by a physician; however, it is dangerous to diagnose yourself; you could have an abscess around the anal opening, and this will not resolve itself.

QUESTION: What is the difference between external and internal hemorrhoids?

ANSWER: The improper answer would be to say that an internal hemorrhoid is inside and an external hemorrhoid is outside. Many times a patient has such large internal hemorrhoids that they are protruding outside, so this answer would be wrong. The proper answer is that internal hemorrhoids are covered by rectal mucosa (lining of the rectum), while external hemorrhoids are covered by skin.

QUESTION: Is it important to know the difference between internal and external hemorrhoids?

ANSWER: Yes, because the lining of the rectum, which covers the internal hemorrhoids, has absolutely no feeling to it at all, and of course the skin that covers the external hemorrhoids has the same feeling as the skin of the rest of your body.

QUESTION: How far does skin go up inside the anal canal?

ANSWER: Skin from the buttocks goes up into the anal canal about one-half to three-quarters of an inch.

QUESTION: How important is it to know that internal hemorrhoids have no feeling and external hemorrhoids have feeling?

ANSWER: It is important to know because if a person has bright red bleeding and no pain, then the bleeding can easily be diagnosed as coming from the internal hemorrhoids rather than the external hemorrhoids. Further discussion of painless bleeding may be found in the chapter on cancer.

QUESTION: If any complication of external hemorrhoids occurs, should there be pain?

ANSWER: Generally, yes. Because the external hemorrhoids are covered by skin, any complications such as a tear, abscess, or blood clot (thrombotic hemorrhoid) will cause pain.

QUESTION: When should a person have a hemorrhoidectomy?

ANSWER: A patient should have a hemorrhoidectomy when the hemorrhoids are giving enough problems that it is worth going through the surgery. You do not have a hemorrhoidectomy just because you have large hemorrhoids. I had one patient who wanted a hemorrhoidectomy so he could get even with his health insurance company for his paying twenty years of premiums and never having been sick.

QUESTION: Is it dangerous to continually bleed off and on from your hemorrhoids, even though it is bright red blood?

ANSWER: Yes. Bleeding from your hemorrhoids can mask a growth in the colon that may be getting larger, and you will not know that you have a growth there because you think the bleeding is coming from your hemorrhoids.

QUESTION: Does this mean that you can have bright red bleeding from a growth four or five feet up in your colon?

ANSWER: Yes. You can have intermittent bright red bleeding from a growth up in your colon, which can be insidious, just like hemorrhodial bleeding; thus, it is extremely dangerous to continually bleed from your hemorrhoids.

QUESTION: Then is it a myth that upper colon bleeding has to be dark and rectal bleeding has to be bright red?

ANSWER: Yes, this is a myth, because many times upper colon bleeding can be bright red and will appear exactly the same as rectal bleeding or hemorrhoidal bleeding.

QUESTION: How serious is a hemorrhoidectomy?

ANSWER: Well, the old cliché is: if the operation is done on you, it is minor; if it is done on me, it is major. However, nowadays, with refined techniques, 95 percent of my patients have their hemorrhoidectomy done as an outpatient. They go in in the morning, have the surgery (which takes approximately thirty to forty-five minutes), and then go home that afternoon. But don't get me wrong—any operation that requires a general or spinal anesthetic is serious; however, so is driving a car.

QUESTION: If you work outside the home on an eight-hour job, approximately how long would you be off work following your hemorrhoidectomy?

ANSWER: My average patient is usually off work approximately seven days; however, there are exceptions. Some will go back to work in four or five days, and other patients will stay off work two weeks.

QUESTION: What activities can I do at home postoperatively?

ANSWER: Unlike a gallbladder operation or an appendectomy, a hemorrhoidectomy is not an incapacitating operation, and a patient may do almost anything around the house that he or she wishes. Patients react to pain and operations in different ways. One time I did a hemorrhoidectomy on a psychiatrist, and when I went by to see him the next morning I asked him how he spent the night. "Praying for death," was his answer.

QUESTION: What should one do when a patient suddenly develops pain in the anal and perianal area?

ANSWER: One should seek out a physician for help, because the pain could be due to a variety of problems, such as thrombotic hemorrhoids, acute fissure in ano, or even an acute fistula in ano (abscess of the anus). Some anal and perianal problems, if not treated immediately, can become very serious in a relatively short period of time (twenty-four to forty-eight hours).

QUESTION: Is it a mistake to try to push a thrombotic hemorrhoid back into the anal canal (or rectum)?

ANSWER: Yes. Very commonly a patient will try to push the external clot back into the rectum to try to get relief, thinking that the knot has protruded from inside. This maneuver will only cause more pain, and usually the knot will come right back out of the rectum.

QUESTION: Can a patient with large prolapsing internal hemorrhoids cause damage by cleaning too vigorously after a bowel movement?

ANSWER: Yes. If a patient prolapses his internal hemorrhoids with each bowel movement, he can do a lot of damage to the delicate rectal lining with vigorous wiping with toilet tissue.

Chapter IV

Fissure in Ano

QUESTION: What is a fissure?

ANSWER: A fissure is a split, tear, or crack in the skin portion of the anal canal. Fissures usually occur just inside the anal opening.

QUESTION: Since a fissure is usually on the skin side of the anal canal, does this mean that a fissure is painful?

ANSWER: Yes. A fissure can be very painful, especially with bowel movements, and this discomfort can last for hours after a bowel movement.

QUESTION: What causes a fissure?

ANSWER: Many times a fissure is caused by a patient's eating too many high residue food products, such as milk, cheese, ice cream, chocolates, et cetera; however, if a patient gets so busy that he forgets to have a bowel movement for several days, this too can cause a fissure. In other words, a fissure is caused by the diameter of the stool being larger than the diameter of the anal opening.

QUESTION: Does this mean that people should not eat high residue products?

ANSWER: No. Patients may eat high residue products, but they should eat them in moderation, mixed in with low residue products.

QUESTION: Explain more about high residue food products.

ANSWER: I find in my practice that people who have gone on milk, cheese, ice cream, and chocolate binges are more likely to develop fissures in the anal canal. These products are more likely to produce a large stool, which is hard to pass. Once a fissure develops, it is hard to heal, because you can't stop having bowel movements while it heals.

QUESTION: What are some of the do's and don'ts if you have a fissure?

ANSWER: One should definitely not hold back from trying to have a bowel movement or try to miss several days so that he will not experience the pain of a bowel movement. Also, one should not take laxatives, because this may tend to give the person loose bowels or diarrhea, which will be severely painful, almost like throwing acid on a cut.

QUESTION: What can a person do at home to alleviate the discomfort of a fissure in ano before seeing the doctor?

ANSWER: Whether the fissure be an acute episode or a chronic fissure (ulcer), the first thing the person should do is to omit all high residue food products from his diet for at least three weeks. The patient may also use a mild stool softener as long as the softener does not make the stool semiliquid or watery. Also, sitting in warm water several times a day will alleviate the discomfort.

QUESTION: What can a doctor do in his office as an office procedure to help heal a fissure?

ANSWER: The doctor may cauterize the fissure with silver nitrate or may inject a long-lasting anesthetic into the tissues beneath the fissure, which will in 85 percent of patients heal the fissure, but it may not be long-lasting.

QUESTION: Is surgery always necessary if a patient has a fissure?

ANSWER: No. There are means of curing a fissure with conservative treatment rather than surgery. Usually an acute fissure will respond to the above treatment, as well as suppositories, ointments, and a low-residue diet.

QUESTION: In what cases is it necessary to operate on a fissure?

ANSWER: If a patient has had a fissure for several months or years and it is chronically inflamed and infected and gives the appearance of an ulceration, this type of fissure usually will benefit from minor surgery. Usually if a fissure does not respond in a few weeks or months to conservative means, then surgery is indicated. If left untreated, it is not rare for a chronic fissure to develop an abscess (fistula in ano).

QUESTION: Explain minor surgery as to length of time in the hospital and time off work.

ANSWER: With our newer modern techniques in surgery, fissurectomies are commonly done on an outpatient basis, and the patient is in the hospital or surgical center just for a few hours and is under anesthesia for twenty to thirty minutes. Patients usually stay home three or four days if they have a job outside the home and may do almost any work at home they feel up to doing while they are recuperating.

QUESTION: What are the symptoms and signs of a fissure?

ANSWER: A patient will have pain when he has a bowel movement, and this pain may last for several minutes to several hours following his bowel movement. He may also have bleeding, which shows up on the side of the stool or is seen on the toilet tissue or drips in the commode. This type of bleeding is usually bright red in nature and usually stops as soon as the bowel movement is over. The patient usually has to strain to have a bowel movement because of the high residue products he has eaten.

QUESTION: If this patient does not seek medical help for his fissure, what will his symptoms be like over two or three months?

ANSWER: With this patient's bowel movements he will have increased pain, which will be intermittent. By this I mean that he may have pain with his bowel movement one day and then will go two days without any pain, and then he may have pain for three days in a row. This is because he tends to eat more high residue foods on certain days than on other days, which reflect on the diameter of his bowel movement and the amount of discomfort he has with a bowel movement.

QUESTION: What is the difference between high residue food products and low residue food products, and give some examples.

ANSWER: A high residue food product means that when the body gets through with using all of the nutrients that it wants in the food that has been digested, the residue from this food product is high, meaning that there will be a lot of waste material. A low residue product means that no matter how much you eat of that product, the body will use most of the material and there will be very little waste material, regardless of the amount you eat. Examples of such high residue products are milk, cheese, ice cream, and chocolates. Examples of low residue products are meat, fish, fruits, and vegetables.

QUESTION: Does the size and diameter of the stool depend on how much you eat or what you eat?

ANSWER: A large, voluminous stool usually means that you have been eating high residue food products for the past few days. Large stools do not necessarily mean that you have eaten in great quantities. An infant will have a large bowel movement because of all the milk he drinks each day. Most of the time a large bowel movement will reflect what you ate and not how much you ate.

QUESTION: What are the two essential procedures that a surgeon must do to correct a fissure at the time of surgery so that it will not reoccur?

ANSWER: A surgeon must remove the fissure and must make the opening the proper size, the problem being that the anal opening is too small to pass a stool without splitting the opening.

QUESTION: Why should the surgeon make the anal opening the proper size?

ANSWER: If the surgeon only takes out the fissure and does not enlarge the anal opening (which, by the way, is not cutting of muscle), then the patient has the same diameter to his anal opening as before, and the fissure will reoccur.

QUESTION: Can some weight-reducing food products be harmful to the anal opening and cause fissures?

ANSWER: Yes. The products that contain a lot of cellulose by-products can cause fissures. These cellulose by-products fill you up so you deceive your appetite, but at the same time they are not properly digested by the intestinal tract, and they produce large stools that are difficult to pass.

QUESTION: Are there other ways of producing anal fissures?

ANSWER: In my practice, very uncommon means are anal intercourse and self-inflicted trauma (foreign objects).

QUESTION: Is having a fissure and being homosexual dangerous?

ANSWER: Yes. A fissure of the anus may be one of the portals of entry for the AIDS virus.

Chapter V

Anal Fistula

QUESTION: What is a fistula?

ANSWER: The true medical definition of a fistula is an opening that is on two different epithelial surfaces connected by a channel or sinus tract. As an example, if a patient has a hole on the outside of his cheek and an opening on the lining of his cheek, with a channel that connects the two openings so that a pencil may be placed into the outer opening and will come out through the inner opening, this is a fistula.

QUESTION: What causes anal fistulas?

ANSWER: Most anal fistulas are caused by the anal glands, which are situated in the anal canal at the junction of the anal skin and the beginning of the lining of the rectum, becoming infected from the bacteria in the stool and forming an abscess next to the anal opening.

QUESTION: What are some of the signs and symptoms of a fistula?

29

ANSWER: When a gland in the anal canal gets infected, it forms an abscess next to the rectum, which begins with a dull, aching pain and may be confused with prostate trouble or the constant urge to have a bowel movement. As the abscess becomes larger, so does the pain, and eventually a knot will appear next to the anal opening that is very tender and not unlike a boil. If a patient can stand it long enough, the boil will rupture, draining pus and giving the patient relief. If the abscess is large enough, it can inhibit urinating and can cause chills and fever.

QUESTION: If the abscess of a fistula empties and drains, does this mean that the fistula goes away forever?

ANSWER: No, the fistula usually comes back in either several days, several weeks, or several months.

QUESTION: Why is a fistula not cured if it drains?

ANSWER: The fistula is not cured because the primary opening, or gland in the anal canal that became infected, continues to become infected because of the bacteria in the stool; thus, the fistula continues to recur.

QUESTION: Are antibiotics the treatment of choice in an acute fistula in ano with an abscess?

ANSWER: No. The treatment of choice is surgery, and antibiotics will not cure a fistula.

QUESTION: Explain surgery as a treatment of choice if a patient has a fistula.

ANSWER: Again, most of the time a fistulectomy is done on an outpatient basis. The patient goes to the hospital one morning, is given an anesthetic for thirty or forty minutes, and when fully awake and alert may go home.

QUESTION: Do fistulas recur?

ANSWER: Fistulas usually recur if the primary opening, that is, the opening inside the anal canal, is not removed. If the surgeon does not remove the primary opening of a fistula and merely incises and drains the abscess, the fistula will recur.

QUESTION: I have heard of some people losing control of their sphincter muscles after a fistulectomy; is this true?

ANSWER: A fistulectomy can be a very delicate operation, and in the hands of a specialist, a patient should not lose any muscle control; however, if the fistula is improperly removed, some of the sphincter muscles can be cut and a patient can lose control.

QUESTION: If a fistula can be a painful knot and a thrombotic hemorrhoid can be a painful knot, both adjacent to the anal opening, how can one tell the difference?

ANSWER: It is very difficult, and most patients cannot tell the difference until it is too late. A thrombotic hemorrhoid occurs almost instantaneously and in the first day has the most pain, with the pain decreasing over the next three to five days until no more pain is felt. A fistula starts with a mild pain, and the discomfort and swelling increase over the next two or three days until the pain is unbearable; then the abscess either empties and gives relief or the patient seeks medical help and the doctor either drains or removes the abscess.

QUESTION: Does the abscess of a fistula grow rapidly?

ANSWER: Yes. The abscess can double every twenty-four hours, so it is prudent to seek medical help as soon as possible.

QUESTION: Are there different types of fistula in the anal and rectal region?

ANSWER: Yes. There is a fistula called a submucosal fistula, which instead of protruding out toward the skin goes up along the side wall of the rectum and is very difficult to diagnose and treat.

QUESTION: Are there other causes of fistulas besides an infected anal gland?

ANSWER: Yes. There can be foreign bodies such as swallowed chicken bones or open safety pins that can cause a rectal fistula. Foreign objects that are placed up into the anal canal and break can also cause an infection with ensuing abscess formation.

QUESTION: Are fistula abscesses different from other types of abscesses on the body?

ANSWER: Yes. A fistula in the region of the anal opening can become very large and usually does not become systemic in nature. By this I mean that the infection does not get into the bloodstream, causing chills and fever. The perianal part of the body has an excellent defense mechanism of encapsulating the abscess and most of the time keeping the infection in that area, as opposed to an abscess in other parts of the body that might become systemic, giving a person chills and fever and making the entire body sick. Anal fistula abscesses are not cured by simple drainage alone, while most abscesses in other parts of the body are cured by drainage.

QUESTION: Is it common for a patient with a fistula not to be able to urinate?

ANSWER: Yes, this is very common. In fact, some patients come to me with the chief complaint that they cannot urinate, and upon examination they are found to have an anal fistula abscess.

QUESTION: How long does a patient usually stay off work after a fistula operation?

ANSWER: This depends on whether the patient comes to the doctor early or comes to the doctor late. If the patient comes to the doctor early, with a small abscessed fistula, then the time off work is only about three or four days. If the patient waits four to six days to seek medical help, then the incision to cure the fistula is larger and the patient may need to stay off work as long as two weeks.

QUESTION: In your opinion, what is the most symptomatic fistula to have and the most difficult on which to operate?

ANSWER: The rectovaginal fistula. This fistula is commonly caused by either an episiotomy or a colonic disease such as chronic ulcerative colitis.

QUESTION: Why are these fistulas so miserable for the patient?

ANSWER: These fistulas consist of an opening in the rectum and an opening in the vagina connected by a channel. Stool and gas from the rectum can escape through the fistula and come out of the vagina at will. The patient has no way to keep from soiling or from preventing the escape of gas through the vagina. Many a woman has had difficulty trying to keep a marriage alive when she can't do her homework.

QUESTION: Is it a difficult operation to repair a rectovaginal fistula?

ANSWER: Yes. Those created by chronic ulcerative colitis are almost impossible to repair because of the diseased tissue. Those problems caused by episiotomies are less difficult to repair and usually have a better than 90 percent chance of success.

QUESTION: Is it true that sometimes a colostomy has to be part of the repair of a rectovaginal fistula?

ANSWER: Yes. It is not uncommon to perform a colostomy to divert the fecal stream so that the fistula repair can heal properly.

Chapter VI

Constipation

QUESTION: What is constipation?

ANSWER: Constipation can be defined in many ways. Constipation may be defined as the inability to pass a large stool that is in the rectum. Another definition is the inability to have a bowel movement whether there is any stool in the rectum or not. Another definition is the inability to have a bowel movement every day. Other definitions include having to take laxatives all the time, having straining and/or bleeding with each bowel movement, and not passing enough stool to satisfy oneself.

QUESTION: Is there a difference between male and female when it comes to bowel habits?

ANSWER: Yes, there is quite a bit of difference. Generally, ninety-nine out of one hundred men will have a bowel movement every day and sometimes twice a day, without any help; however, ninety-nine out of one hundred females will have a bowel movement every two or three days, and it is not uncommon for the female to have a bowel movement once a week.

QUESTION: Why is there this difference in male and female bowel habits?

ANSWER: The colon in the female is larger and can store more waste material. Also, the waste material is much drier, because while it is being stored, more water is being drawn out of the waste material. The male colon is smaller than the female colon and therefore cannot store as much waste material, and consequently passes a more watery, semiliquid stool, as opposed to the dry, firm stool that the female passes.

QUESTION: Is a person supposed to have a bowel movement every day to stay healthy?

ANSWER: No. A person does not have to have a bowel movement every day to stay healthy. If a person's regularity is once a day, then that is fine; however, if a person's regularity is every three or four days, or once a week, that is also fine and does not inhibit good health.

QUESTION: Since most females have a bowel movement every two or three days or once a week, isn't this frustrating to the female as she grows up knowing her brother or her husband has a bowel movement every day and sometimes twice a day without the use of any laxatives or dietary means?

ANSWER: Yes, this is very frustrating to the female because in most families the mother has instilled in the children that a bowel movement every day is healthy, which only frustrates the female more; then, when she gets married and her husband has a bowel movement every day, if not twice a day, many times she resorts to laxatives and special diets in order to have a bowel movement every day, such as he does.

QUESTION: Does promptly answering the urge to have a bowel movement help in avoiding constipation?

ANSWER: Yes. In the male, the urge to have a bowel movement is one of the only signals that the brain interprets from the perineal area, and thus when a male gets the urge to have a bowel movement, he generally responds immediately to the urge. The female gets many sensations from the perineal and pelvic area, including those caused by menstrual cycles, postmentrual syndrome, or douching, and thus the urge to have a bowel movement is not as significant in the female as it is in the male. It is easier for the female to put off having a bowel movement and not answer the urge. Most females must be tranquil in order to have a bowel movement and must not be preoccupied with getting the children off to school, making sure her husband is not late for work, and making sure that the telephone does not ring.

QUESTION: Does a female have a more difficult bowel movement than the male?

ANSWER: Yes. In general, since the colon is larger and has more inner surface area, more water is drawn out of the female stool; thus, the female must pass a much larger and drier stool. Since the male colon is smaller and cannot store as much waste material, the male has an easier time of passing the stool because it is smaller and more moist.

QUESTION: Why do most doctors say that you must drink eight glasses of water a day to improve your regularity?

ANSWER: One of the main functions of the colon is to supply the body cells with fluid; thus, the fluid is drawn from the inside of the colon and is passed on to the body tissues. If a person drinks an adequate amount of fluids each day, some of this liquid will supply the body cells, leaving some liquid in the colon to moisten the stool, making it easier to pass.

QUESTION: If you eat some chicken today, is the waste material that you pass tomorrow necessarily that same chicken?

ANSWER: No, it is probably not. The chicken that you eat today may not pass as waste material for two or three days.

QUESTION: What is the transit time of food through the gastrointestinal tract from the time it is eaten until the time it is expelled?

ANSWER: After you eat a typical piece of chicken, the chicken will be assimilated in the stomach and small intestines, which is approximately twenty-five feet of intestinal tract, in approximately thirty minutes. The waste material, still being in liquid form, will leave the small intestine and enter the right side of the colon and will then traverse around the colon. All materials that are beneficial to the body have been extracted from the food product within the thirty minutes that it takes to travel through the small intestines. The waste material, which is liquid, is then ready to travel through the colon for storage. This transit through the colon may take two or three days to occur, even though some food products in a person may traverse the entire large and small intestines (thirty feet) in just two or three hours.

QUESTION: Since most men have a bowel movement every day and sometimes twice a day, is it true that there are very few food products that will make a man constipated?

ANSWER: True. There are very few products that will make a man constipated; however, the most common food products that will tend to make a man constipated, if he goes on binges with them, are milk and milk products such as cheese, ice cream, and chocolates. If a man is constipated or thinks he is constipated, it takes very little help from a stool softener or from bran each morning to regulate him.

QUESTION: Can a female get constipated more easily than a man?

ANSWER: Most females feel as if they are constipated all the time, regardless of what they eat or what they pass. Since the majority of females have a bowel movement only every two or three days and because they have to strain so hard in order to have that bowel movement, they naturally feel they are constipated. If a female passes only small little pellets of stool and has to strain to do that, she feels she is constipated, not realizing that the consistency of a person's stool has to do with what he or she eats. If a female does not feel good any particular day and has a headache with bloating and a lot of gas, she will attribute this to being constipated and to not having a "good" bowel movement for a day or so.

QUESTION: Are laxatives good for you?

ANSWER: Laxatives, if used wisely, can be of immense help. A good example of this is if a person takes a car trip for four or five days and gets off schedule and cannot get relief from a small enema, then a one-time laxative will give the patient relief, and in this case a laxative is useful.

QUESTION: Can laxatives be habit-forming?

ANSWER: Yes. Laxatives can be habit-forming because they not only mess up your regular bowel habits, but they mess up your thinking in regard to your bowel habits.

QUESTION: How can laxatives mess up your bowel habits?

ANSWER: Well, if a person takes a laxative, it will empty the entire small intestine as well as the entire large intestine. After a person takes a laxative and the entire gastrointestinal tract is empty, and a person eats again, it obviously will take two to four days for the intestinal tract to become full again so that the waste material reaches the rectum and the patient will again get the urge to have a bowel movement, approximately on the third or fourth day or longer.

QUESTION: Won't the patient eventually get an urge to have a bowel movement and then start his regular bowel movement?

ANSWER: Most of the time patients who take laxatives do not understand that it takes a certain amount of time to fill up the colon before they can have another bowel movement, and they will become anxious before this time and will repeat the laxative.

QUESTION: What will happen when they repeat the laxative? Is this how they get on a laxative habit?

ANSWER: Yes; they repeat the laxative before it is time for them to have a normal bowel movement. Naturally, they have a fairly good bowel movement because they have cleaned themselves out again and they think they feel better. Now that they have to start the entire process over again, are they going to wait until they begin to have normal bowel movements or are they going to get so nervous after the third or fourth day that they again reach for the laxative bottle?

QUESTION: What is another reason that people like to take laxatives?

ANSWER: Another reason that people like to take laxatives is because they pass so much more than they would normally pass having a regular bowel movement, and their psyche tells them that they feel better that day and that they have more strength because they have passed more. Another reason they feel better is that they feel they have emptied out the colon and thus they will not absorb the toxic elements that would have been left in the colon, which of course is completely a myth. Another reason is that they pass a lot of gas taking a laxative and are not quite as bloated as they might normally be. This also gives them a feeling of well-being, and so they continue to take laxatives. Some people who have whipped their colon feel you must take a laxative to have a bowel movement because the colon becomes lazy and worn-out like a tired mule, but these people are usually in their seventies, eighties, or nineties, and not in their forties, fifties, or sixties.

QUESTION: Can regular-sized enemas then also be habit-forming?

ANSWER: Yes. Regular-sized enemas, a quart or two of water, will go up the rectum and grab two or three days' worth of bowel movement; thus, the patient, after having taken an enema, must realize that it will take again two or three days to get back to his normal, regular routine; however, most patients, having seen how much they can pass with an enema and feeling a false sense of well-being after taking an enema, continue to take enemas, feeling that they want to empty out their entire colon so that no toxins can be released into the body from any waste material that is left in the colon.

QUESTION: If a person thinks he is constipated, how can he regulate himself?

43

ANSWER: I have found out in my private practice that if a patient has been on laxatives or has taken enemas for years, if he follows certain instructions that I give him, he will slowly become regular and will get off of laxatives and enemas.

QUESTION: What are these instructions that you have given your patients?

ANSWER: First, I tell them to get a four ounce infant syringe; this can be obtained at most drugstores; then, I have them make out a chart. In the first column, they put down the days. In the second column, they put down *yes* or *no* as to the fact that they have given themselves a little four ounce enema that day. In the third column, they put down the results, which will be either a plus or a 0; they do not have to describe in any manner the results. During this three-week period they do not take any laxatives or enemas. Each day they give themselves a four ounce syringe of warm tap water at any time of the day. If they pass any amount of stool, no matter what the amount, for that twenty-four hours they put a plus in the third column. If they do not have to pass any waste material for that twenty-four hours, they put a 0 in the column. They do not have to pass the waste material or have a bowel movement at the same time they give themselves the syringe. They can give themselves the syringe full of water at 7:00 in the morning without results, and if they have a bowel movement at noon, this counts as a plus in the third column.

QUESTION: Will this help them regulate themselves?

ANSWER: Yes. This will not only help them regulate themselves but this will also tell the person when they are truly supposed to have a bowel movement, whether it be every day, every other day, every third day, et cetera.

QUESTION: Is this easy for the patient to do?

ANSWER: No, it is very difficult for patients to do because when they follow these instructions, they have usually just taken a large dose of laxative or a large enema, so they will get several zeros in the days following the time they have seen you at the office and will become panicked and want to take an enema or a laxative; however, if you can instill confidence in patients regarding leaving off the laxatives and enemas, and let them realize that when they start having their normal bowel movements they will not be passing as much as they did using the laxatives and enemas, they will eventually change their way of thinking and change their bowel habits. Some people have the funny idea that the more stool they pass each day, the more strength they have that day.

QUESTION: What will the chart show after three weeks?

ANSWER: The chart after three weeks will show patients that, not having taken laxatives or enemas, do have a bowel movement every so often. This is shown by the third column, because most people who have a normal bowel movement will empty out only the last eight to ten inches of the colon, and thus, using the little syringe, the small amount of four ounces of warm tap water will also empty out just the lower eight to ten inches of colon, which is normal for a person. Let me emphasize again that you do not have to have a bowel movement every day to be healthy.

QUESTION: Will the patient have to use this four ounce syringe all the time?

ANSWER: No. After a month or two, patients will realize that they are supposed to have so much bowel movement evacuated on a certain day, and they will then get their confidence back so that they do not have to use the enema, and they will then start getting the urge on that particular day and will pass the stool in the lower eight to ten inches of the colon. They will also be happy regardless, even though they do not pass as large an amount of waste material as they did when they took an enema or laxatives.

QUESTION: What are colonic lavages, and are they good for you?

ANSWER: Colonic lavage is giving a patient multiple high so-called colonic enemas that completely evacuate the entire colon, in a clinic or simulated clinic, usually in somebody's home. This, again, makes the patient psychologically feel that he has emptied all of the toxins in his colon, and that he will feel better because he will not have to absorb these toxins; of course, this is one of the myths about the colon that is totally wrong.

QUESTION: Is there any danger in colonic lavages?

ANSWER: Yes. If the colonic lavage is not properly administered and the patient has not had a proper history and physical examination, a colonic lavage can perforate the colon or do some damage to some preexisting disease in the colon. The water can also be too hot and can burn the inner lining of the colon. If the enema tips and instruments are not properly sterilized, certain venereal diseases such as herpes, gonorrhea, and warts can be transmitted to the patient. It has recently been felt that posssibly AIDS can also be transmitted in this manner.

QUESTION: Why are there so many laxatives and stool softeners in the drugstore?

ANSWER: The reason for this is that one laxative usually does not satisfy a person for more than three or four weeks. This is because a person will take a laxative and pass a lot of material; then, in a day or two, he will pass still some more material that is of fairly good size; however, as he continues to take the laxative doses closer and closer together, day in and day out, obviously his gastronintestinal tract is completely empty, and the fact that nothing is produced when he continually takes consecutive laxatives makes him feel that the laxative is not working; thus, he will go to the drugstore and find another laxative that may work better.

QUESTION: Are stool softeners and laxatives essentially the same thing?

ANSWER: Yes. Stool softeners are a mild form of laxative. Whereas a laxative is considered to be a medication taken if severe constipation is present, a stool softener is taken daily to give some aid in the daily passage of the person's bowel movement.

QUESTION: Will bran each morning for breakfast help regulate a person's bowel movements?

ANSWER: Yes. Bran, a high residue food product, will aid most people in having regular bowel movements, but may also cause a flare-up of certain diseases such as chronic ulcerative colitis and diverticulitis.

QUESTION: Does constipation give a person a lot of bloating and gas, headaches, and bad breath?

ANSWER: Constipation will rarely give a patient any of those symptoms; this is merely a myth. Bloating and gas formation are mainly caused by chewing gum, smoking, air swallowing, drinking cold liquids, drinking liquids through straws, certain food products, and belching. The headache you have that day could be because you have been chewed out or you found out that your wife was having an affair, and the bad breath could be due either to poor oral hygiene, organic oral pathology, or sinus infection. Very rarely, if ever, are these symptoms due to constipation.

QUESTION: Which type of bowel movement, constipation or diarrhea, will generally bring on more types of complication seen by a proctologist year in and year out?

ANSWER: In my practice, diarrhea will cause complications 80 percent more times than will constipation, in the average patient.

QUESTION: Is it very hard and time-consuming to regulate a person who has been a long-time laxative user or enema user?

ANSWER: Yes. It usually takes three or four times longer to solve a problem such as this, because a patient has certain myths and conclusions already established in his mind, and most of them cannot be broken with just one visit; it may take three or four visits, and even then their doctor may not succeed in getting a patient off of laxatives. I have often joked that I can take a person's hemorrhoids out faster than I can get a person off of laxatives.

QUESTION: Tell me about the syndrome called "coccydynia" or "levator muscle spasm."

ANSWER: This occurs in women 99 percent more than in men. It is a condition giving patients (mainly the female) a feeling of fullness or pressure in the lower rectum by the tailbone. Patients think they are constipated and run to the bathroom all day trying to pass a stool that isn't there. This feeling is produced by a muscle that is attached to the tailbone and flares out to each buttock. This muscle is called the levator muscle. When it goes into spasm due to nervousness and tension, it causes a dull, aching pain in the lower rectum that the patient interprets as being constipated. In trying to get rid of this feeling, she will take laxatives or enemas and will strain all day on the commode, trying to pass a muscle spasm.

QUESTION: What kind of stress or nervousness brings on this levator spasm?

ANSWER: Usually these problems are irreversible or insoluble. I can but illustrate with examples: mother-in-law living with you, husband takes early retirement and follows his wife around the house all day, husband drinks too much whiskey, son on drugs, et cetera. It is usually some problem the female cannot immediately solve, and her levator muscle is the target organ. Levator muscle spasms are second cousins to tension headaches, spastic colon, and stomach ulcers.

Chapter VII

Diarrhea

QUESTION: What is the definition of diarrhea?

ANSWER: Diarrhea has many definitions. It can be (1) loose bowel movements; it can be (2) multiple watery, loose bowel movements; it can be (3) multiple bowel movements per day if the person is just used to one bowel movement each day.

QUESTION: What causes diarrhea?

ANSWER: Diarrhea is merely a symptom of an underlying disease. Diarrhea can be caused by a multitude of things, including anything from diet to disease.

QUESTION: What are some of the common causes of diarrhea?

ANSWER: Some of the common causes of diarrhea fall into the dietary category. Certain dietary products such as fresh fruit or fresh vegetables, highly seasoned foods, or nuts will give a patient diarrhea if eaten either in small quantities or large quantities. Other more subtle products that can be eaten and will give diarrhea can be vitamins

51

with iron in them, isolated products such as coconut or chocolate, or a variety of other specific food products. Food products that give one person diarrhea may not give it to another person.

QUESTION: How can a patient find out what food product gives him diarrhea?

ANSWER: Diarrhea from a food product can be brought on almost immediately within thirty to sixty minutes or can be brought on within twenty-four hours; thus, a patient must play detective and figure out what food product he ate, within the twenty-four hours prior to the onset of the diarrhea, that most likely caused it.

QUESTION: What else causes diarrhea in a patient?

ANSWER: Another thing that may cause diarrhea in a patient is the ingestion of a foreign bacteria or a virus. Common diseases of this nature are Salmonella, Shigella, and botulism, which are certain types of food poisoning.

QUESTION: How quickly will these bacteria and viruses make a person sick?

ANSWER: Again, depending on each individual person, these diseases may make a person sick within two hours or within six to eight hours.

QUESTION: How harmful are these common food poisonings to a patient?

ANSWER: They may be very harmful if not fatal to the very young or very old person, but generally they produce only harsh symptoms in most people; however, botulism is a definite poisoning and may be lethal to most people. People who go to a foreign country and get diarrhea with vomiting for several days may be so miserable that they wish they had died, however.

QUESTION: Can a patient keep from getting diarrhea if he is going to a foreign country?

ANSWER: A patient may take certain antibiotics starting twenty-four hours prior to departure, which may prevent him from getting diarrhea; however, this is not 100 percent sure. There are some excellent medications on the market that will control the diarrhea, once a patient obtains it. Definitely take some medication to control diarrhea on a trip so you won't ruin any sightseeing excursions.

QUESTION: Why is it so important to stop diarrhea, once a person obtains it?

ANSWER: It is important to stop the diarrhea or at least control it because several complications can occur from the continuation of diarrhea.

QUESTION: What are these complications given to a patient by diarrhea?

ANSWER: These complications can be a flare-up of your hemorrhoids in the form of thrombotic hemorrhoids or blood clots, which is very common in diarrhea. It is not rare for diarrhea to get an anal gland infected, producing an acute fistula in ano. Diarrhea may also produce severe anal and perianel irritation and itching, which can be hard to control.

QUESTION: Is it easier for the male or for the female to acquire diarrhea?

ANSWER: It is uncommon in the female to get diarrhea in the usual manner (dietary, et cetera) unless she has some underlying disease, or unless she has obtained food poisoning. It is very common for the male to get diarrhea because most males are already very regular and have one if not two bowel movements a day. If the male eats anything such as fresh fruit or fresh vegetables or highly seasoned foods in excess or on a consecutive basis, it is not uncommon for him to have diarrhea. These food products can easily increase his gastrointestinal transit time, which is already very regular.

QUESTION: When should a patient go to a doctor for diarrhea?

QUESTION: A patient should seek medical help if the diarrhea is persistent for several hours or if the patient passes any bloody diarrhea or bloody mucus with his diarrhea. He should also seek immediate help if he has cramping abdominal pain, nausea, or vomiting.

QUESTION: Why is bloody diarrhea or bloody mucus so important as to require that medical help be sought immediately?

54

ANSWER: Bloody diarrhea or bloody mucus means that the diarrhea has caused enough irritation of the gastrointestinal tract to erode into blood vessels in the lining of the colon. A tumor, unknown up to this point, can be irritated enough that the surface may start bleeding, or a completely new disease may have occurred such as chronic ulcerative colitis or diverticulitis.

QUESTION: In what ways can diarrhea affect the body?

ANSWER: Diarrhea, if it is prolonged, can cause dehydration, which can upset many bodily functions. Dehydration in the very young or infant, or in the very old, can be very devastating and should be treated immediately. The average patient can handle diarrhea and dehydration fairly well if his intake matches or exceeds his daily output; therefore, a person with diarrhea should increase his fluids and try to maintain some type of dietary intake. Years ago, before sterile needles and sterile intravenous solutions were available, dehydration was treated by giving the patient water enemas. The colon would completely absorb the water from the enemas and supply the body cells as needed.

QUESTION: How does dehydration occur in diarrhea?

ANSWER: The transit time of the waste material in the gastrointestinal tract is so rapid that the colon does not have time to absorb the fluid out of the waste material and thus cannot hydrate the body cells. The ratio is upset and more fluid is being lost through the rectum than is being absorbed for the body cells.

QUESTION: What causes the extreme irritation in the anal and perianel area in diarrhea?

ANSWER: The transit time in the gastrointestinal tract is so fast that the enzymes and acids that are produced in the stomach, pancreas, and gallbladder are not broken down into their basic elements and thus hit the anal and perianel area in their natural state, which is extremely irritating to the anal and perianal skin, which does not have the protective mechanism that the lining of the rectum has.

QUESTION: How do you treat the anal and perianel irritation caused by diarrhea?

ANSWER: First, find out the cause of the diarrhea and treat the underlying disease; then, try to stop the diarrhea by using certain medications that will control the diarrhea. Third, treat the local area by keeping it dry, cleansing the anal and perianel area with witch hazel, and using baby powder or cornstarch in the area, along with soft cotton pledgets changed every two or three hours to keep the area dry. Also, a mild hydrocortisone cream applied to the anal and perianel area would help the situation. It's just like treating diaper rash—you must keep the area dry. Do not use overkill treatment with a bunch of over-the-counter medications, and keep soap off the area completely.

Chapter VIII

Cancer of the Colon and Rectum

QUESTION: What is a cancer?

ANSWER: A cancer is an abnormal fast growth of cells in the body, which if left alone will eventually destroy good tissue and lead to death.

QUESTION: Is there much cancer of the colon and rectum in the United States?

ANSWER: Cancer of the colon and rectum is the third leading killer of humans in the United States, behind heart disease and cancer of the lung.

QUESTION: How many people in the United States die of cancer of the colon and rectum each year?

ANSWER: Cancer of the colon and rectum in the United States has reached epidemic proportions, with over one hundred thousand people a year dying of cancer of the colon and rectum in the United States. This is not how many have it; this is how many die from it.

QUESTION: I know the colon and rectum is five feet long and is the last part of the gastrointestinal tract, but where in the colon does this cancer occur?

ANSWER: True, the colon/rectum is five feet long; 50 percent of cancers of the colon and rectum occur in the lower rectum, in approximately the lower five inches of the rectum; 75 percent of the cancers of the colon and rectum occur within the lower ten inches of the rectum; and the other 25 percent of the cancers occur above the lower ten inches in the remainder of the colon.

QUESTION: Does this mean that almost half of the people that are going to die of cancer of the colon and rectum could have been saved if they had just had a digital examination by their doctor?

ANSWER: Yes. A digital examination yearly will detect approximately 50 percent of all cancers of the colon and rectum. Of the one hundred thousand people who will die from colon and rectal cancer this year, approximately fifty percent would have been saved if they would have had a digital examination done by their doctor. If the tumor is detected early by this means, many lives can be saved.

QUESTION: How can the other cancers of the colon and rectum be detected?

ANSWER: The American Cancer Society says that everyone over the age of forty should have a proctoscopic examination once a year. A proctoscope, or proctosigmoidoscope, is a ten-inch (25 cm) metal tube with a light on it that views the lower ten inches of the rectum under direct vision. This is where approximately 75 percent of all cancers of the colon and rectum occur. If the one hundred thousand people that are going to die this year from cancer of the colon and rectum had a proctoscopic examination done, approximately seventy five thousand of those patients would be saved. This examination takes about three to five minutes in a doctor's office and requires no preparation. If the doctor cannot see because of stool in your rectum, then the nurse can give you a fast Fleet enema.

QUESTION: Why does a physician examine the colon above the ten-inch level?

ANSWER: A physician does a colon X ray or colonoscopy examination if the patient has had blood mixed in the stool, a change in bowel habits, unusual cramping abdominal pains, or a strong history of cancer of the colon and rectum in his family. There are other reasons for checking the upper colon; however, those are the most common reasons.

QUESTION: How long does it take in a doctor's office to do a digital examination and a proctosigmoidoscopic examination?

ANSWER: Usually the digital examination and the proctosigmoidoscopic examination take anywhere from three to five minutes. These simple and brief examinations have saved many lives.

QUESTION: What are the two popular ways of checking the upper colon?

ANSWER: One common way of checking the upper colon is by means of colon X rays (lower GI, barium enema). You must prepare your colon the night before the examination. This x-ray examination is done by means of instilling a dye called barium into the rectum, and this contrast medium will flow throughout the entire five feet of colon and will show any abnormal defects in the colon. Sometimes air is put into the colon with the barium, and this is called an air contrast colon X ray. This is done in order to pick up smaller objects such as polyps. The colon X ray is strictly a diagnostic examination; thus, no tumor can be removed and no biopsies can be done. The other common way to examine the upper colon is by means of a colonoscopy examination. You must prepare the colon the night before this examination, also. This examination involves a long five-foot fiberoptic tube, which is flexible, and under direct vision by a specialist, this tube is inserted into the rectum and maneuvered around the entire five feet of colon. If a polyp is present, it can generally be removed by the use of this instrument, and this instrument is also useful in obtaining biopsies of the inner lining of the colon or of various tumors that are seen. There is very little discomfort to it, and most doctors sedate the patient to the point where there is no pain.

QUESTION: Do you need to go into the hospital for these examinations?

ANSWER: The colon X ray can be done either as an outpatient in the hospital or as an outpatient in a radiologist's office, and it takes approximately forty to sixty minutes.

The colonoscopy examination can be done either as an outpatient in the hospital or in an outpatient surgical center, and it usually takes about forty-five minutes to an hour to perform. Both examinations require that the patient prepare his colon the night before. Since the colonoscopy examination is usually done under light sedation, it is required that someone drive you home after a colonoscopy examination.

QUESTION: What is a polyp in the colon?

ANSWER: A polyp is a small growth that is in the shape of a mushroom and is attached to the inner lining of the colon and is generally approximately two centimeters or less in size.

QUESTION: Can these polyps be malignant or turn into a malignancy?

ANSWER: Yes. All polyps that arise from the lining of the colon and rectum can be malignant or can become malignant and should be removed.

QUESTION: In the general population, can most of the polyps that are seen through the colonoscope be removed through the colonoscope?

ANSWER: Yes, most polyps can be removed by using the colonoscope.

ANSWER: What other type of polyp is there?

61

ANSWER: There is also the so-called sessile-type polyp, which is also a growth on the lining of the colon; this does not have a pedicle but has a broad base, as if half a walnut were stuck to the lining. These polyps are more difficult to remove, and some of them cannot be removed at all through the colonoscopy tube.

QUESTION: If a polyp cannot be removed using the colonoscopy tube, does this mean major surgery?

ANSWER: Yes. If a polyp is on a pedicle that is too large to be removed, or if a sessile polyp cannot be removed using the colonoscope, then the portion of colon containing the polyp should be removed by a major surgical resection.

QUESTION: Can some polyps be eventually removed by cauterization with multiple examinations?

ANSWER: Yes. Some smaller polyps can be removed by multiple cauterizations using the colonoscope if they cannot be removed at one time. This would avoid major surgery but is second choice in treatment, and you do run the risk of not knowing what the complete pathology report shows.

QUESTION: If a cancer is detected in the colon and rectum, what is the treatment of choice?

ANSWER: In most cancers of the colon and rectum, the treatment of choice is major radical removal of that portion of the colon that contains the malignancy, including the lymphatic system, which drains that portion of the colon.

QUESTION: Are there certain types of colon and rectal cancers that can be treated and cured by means other than surgery?

ANSWER: Yes, there are certain types of rectal and anorectal cancers that, once biopsied and identified, can be cured by irradiation alone.

QUESTION: Are there several types of cancer of the colon?

ANSWER: Yes, there are several types of cancer of the colon. One type may start in a benign so-called villous tumor and change into a malignancy, and the other arises in the cells lining the colon and is called an adenocarcinoma of the colon. The above-mentioned are the two common types, and if caught early they can be cured.

QUESTION: What mainly determines the cure rate of cancers of the colon and rectum?

ANSWER: The cure rate of cancer of the colon and rectum is mainly determined by the size of the tumor and if it has spread to any of the adjacent structures or lymph nodes or to distant organs.

QUESTION: How does a cancer of the colon and rectum spread in the body?

ANSWER: Colon cancer may spread by the bloodstream, but more commonly will spread through the lymphatic system, which drains the colon and rectum.

QUESTION: Exactly how do most cancers of the colon and rectum spread?

ANSWER: First, the cancer starts growing on the lining of the colon; then, it spreads through the bowel wall. Next, it goes through the lymphatic system to the adjacent lymph nodes and from the lymph nodes it goes to distant organs such as the liver and the lungs.

QUESTION: What determines if a patient has a good chance of survival?

ANSWER: The spread of the tumor determines the survival rate. If the tumor has spread through the bowel wall to the lymph nodes, the survival rate is not as good as if the tumor was just contained to the lining of the bowel, and if the tumor has spread to other organs, then the survival rate becomes even worse, and this patient must be treated with supplemental treatment using chemotherapy or irradiation.

QUESTION: Is irradiation a popular supplement to surgery for cancer of the colon and rectum?

ANSWER: Irradiation used to be popular as an adjunct to most cancers of the colon and rectum, either preoperatively or postoperatively, but recently irradiation has been found to be of little use except in certain anal and perianal cancers.

QUESTION: Is chemotherapy still used as an adjunct to surgery in cancer of the colon and rectum?

ANSWER: Chemotherapy is still used in certain cases of cancer of the colon and rectum, depending on the stage the cancer is in. Chemotherapy is employed usually as a palliative treatment for pain and discomfort, and for longevity.

QUESTION: What is a colostomy?

ANSWER: A colostomy is where a piece of colon is brought up through the abdominal wall and is sewn to the skin as a round, circular opening of the bowel. The person uses the colostomy to eliminate their waste material. There is the permanent colostomy, which a patient has for the rest of his life, and there is the temporary colostomy, which the patient has only for several months.

QUESTION: When is a colostomy necessary?

ANSWER: One good example of the necessity for a colostomy is if a patient has a cancer in the lower rectum, and the lower rectum must be removed completely in order to remove the cancer; then a colostomy must be performed in this patient in order to allow this patient to eliminate his waste material.

QUESTION: Can a person function normally in life with a colostomy?

ANSWER: A colostomy is a small handicap such as wearing glasses, and a person with a colostomy can do practically everything in life that a person without a colostomy can do.

QUESTION: Does a colostomy take a lot of care each day?

ANSWER: No. A colostomy is usually irrigated with tap water each morning for about fifteen to twenty minutes, and then no waste material is eliminated until the next morning, when the irrigation is repeated.

QUESTION: Does this mean that colostomies do not evacuate stool all day long?

ANSWER: That is correct. After a person irrigates his colostomy, the colostomy does not soil for twenty-four hours.

QUESTION: Does a person have to wear a bag on a colostomy every day?

ANSWER: No. In my practice I have many patients who, after they irrigate and wash up, merely tape a piece of Kleenex across the opening of their colostomy; however, most people wear a little plastic bag that cannot be seen under their clothes.

QUESTION: How do people with colostomies take care of any odor or noise that it may produce?

ANSWER: If a person wears a small plastic bag over the opening, usually a couple of charcoal tablets in the bag will take care of the odor, and a small pledget of cotton stuck in the opening will take care of any gas noise.

QUESTION: Are there other types of colosotomy that are not permanent but are only temporary?

ANSWER: Yes. Many so-called double-barrel colostomies are temporary colostomies that are done to divert the fecal stream away from an infected piece of bowel or a piece of bowel that has been operated on and needs to be at rest. After the infection has subsided or the bowel has healed, then the temporary colostomy is replaced back into the abdominal cavity and then the colon functions normally.

QUESTION: Do most cancer operations of the colon and rectum require a colostomy?

ANSWER: No, better than ninety percent of the cancers of the colon and rectum are in such a location that they do not require a colostomy and can be removed by simply moving that portion of the bowel that contains the cancer and joining the bowel back together again without a colostomy.

QUESTION: In doing cancer surgery on the colon and rectum, is it important to take out the lymph nodes in that area that are adjacent to the cancer?

ANSWER: Yes. One of the main ways that a cancer spreads is through the lymphatic system, and when the cancer and the bowel that contains the cancer are removed, the entire lymphatic system draining that area is also removed.

QUESTION: If the cancer of the colon and rectum has spread to the liver or lungs and is just one solitary metastasis, how long should this metastasis be treated?

ANSWER: If it is found that there is just one solitary metastatic lesion that is fairly small in the liver or the lungs, this can be treated surgically by removing this solitary mass, and the patient can also have supplemental chemotherapy.

QUESTION: Does chemotherapy have certain complications in patients?

ANSWER: Chemotherapy in certain patients will have complications. The complications can be lowering of the white count; making the patient very nauseated, with accompanying vomiting; causing a body rash or sore throat; and, last but not least, the loss of hair.

QUESTION: Does irradiation cause any complications when used?

ANSWER: Yes, irradiation can cause cramping abdominal pains. It can also cause nausea and vomiting. It may cause the sloughing of anal and perianal tissue. It can also inhibit and slow up the healing of normal tissue and can cause a lot of skin irritation to the areas that it treats.

QUESTION: Isn't it important to know that cancer of the colon and rectum can easily be cured if caught in time?

ANSWER: If patients would have regular yearly checkups, we would not have the one hundred thousand deaths yearly in the United States that we now have.

QUESTION: What is the first warning of cancer of the colon and rectum?

ANSWER: The first warning of cancer of the colon and rectum is bleeding with your bowel movements. This blood can be bright red or it can be dark blood; it can be continuous blood or it can be occasional bouts of blood every two or three weeks.

QUESTION: What is the myth about the color of blood in cancer of the colon and rectum?

ANSWER: The myth about the blood is that a growth will bleed dark red blood. When a person has cancer of the colon and rectum, the blood does not have to be dark, but can easily be bright red, just like hemorrhoidal bleeding.

QUESTION: Isn't there another myth about cancer of the colon and bleeding?

ANSWER: Yes. This myth about cancer of the colon and rectum is that if you have a tumor, most of the time you hemorrhage, and this is entirely false. The bleeding of the cancer of the colon and rectum is an insidious type of bleeding that mimics hemorrhoidal bleeding, and most of the time a patient cannot tell hemorrhoidal bleeding from cancer bleeding.

QUESTION: Is this why it is so important that any type of rectal bleeding be attended to by a physician?

ANSWER: If a patient waits for the other signs of cancer of the colon and rectum such as change in bowel habits, cramping abdominal pains, anemia, or weight loss, it may be too late for a cure.

QUESTION: Does a surgeon see a patient postoperatively at regular intervals to see if there is any recurrence of the disease or spread of the disease?

ANSWER: Yes. A surgeon will follow a patient at regular intervals postoperatively. The first year to two, he will see the patient more often and will perform and order more tests and X rays than he will in the third, fourth, and fifth years. After the fifth year of survival, you are treated then as any average person.

QUESTION: Is the Hemoccult test done in the doctor's office a good test for cancer of the colon and rectum?

ANSWER: Yes and no. This test is very sensitive and has a large percentage of false positives and false negatives. If a test is positive, the patient must seek further medical care, which is good. If the test is negative, most patients stop there, lulling themselves into complacency and not having any further tests performed.

Chapter IX

Colitis and Diverticulitis

QUESTION: What is colitis?

ANSWER: The definition of colitis is an inflammation of the lining of the colon that can be due to a number of maladies.

QUESTION: Are there many different types of colitis?

ANSWER: Yes. There are as many different types of colitis as there are different types of headaches. When a person says that he has colitis, it could mean a number of things. This statement can be very vague and can mean that this patient has either a very mild disease or a very serious disease of the colon.

QUESTION: What are some of the names of the various types of colitis?

ANSWER: Some of the names of the various types of colitis are spastic colitis, mucus colitis, granulomatous colitis, and chronic ulcerative colitis. There are other different types of colitis that have no specific name, but can be caused by various bacteria, various parasites, or various drugs.

QUESTION: What are some of the more common types of colitis.

ANSWER: Some of the more common types of colitis are those caused by foreign bacteria or parasites that have invaded the intestinal tract, or there can also be types of colitis due to various food products, or psychosomatic colitis.

QUESTION: How can you diagnose which colitis a person has?

ANSWER: First, the physician must take a history and then do a physical examination; then, other specific studies can be done such as obtaining a stool specimen to determine if the patient has picked up any foreign bacteria or parasites. The stool specimen may also be examined for other types of diseases and then, of course, a proctoscopic and possibly a colonoscopic examination should be done and biopsies should be taken. Various other tests may be performed to diagnose rare diseases such as sprue or Whipple's disease of the gastrointestinal tract.

QUESTION: What is mucus colitis and what is usually its cause?

ANSWER: Mucus colitis is when the lining of the colon produces an excessive amount of mucus that is passed and can be seen in the commode mixed with the stool. Some patients can pass small amounts of mucus all day long. The colon normally excretes mucus, but it cannot be seen in the stool. When a person has mucus colitis, then the excessive amount of mucus produced can be identified in the stool or in the commode. Mucus colitis is commonly caused by either certain foods that are ingested or by psychosomatic reasons.

QUESTION: What are some of the common foods that can cause mucus colitis?

ANSWER: Some of the common foods that can cause mucus colitis are certain types of vegetables, certain types of fresh fruit, and certain types of highly seasoned food, especially if they are eaten two or three days in a row. These various food products can be irritating to the lining of the colon, which will cause the lining to produce more mucus, just as placing an onion to one's eye will produce tears. A food product that produces mucus in one person may not produce it in another.

QUESTION: How can psychosomatic problems or functional problems cause mucus colitis?

ANSWER: By means of the autonomic nervous system, which supplies the intestinal tract and over which we have no control. Certain stressful situations, such as the death of a parent or child, or any stressful situation, can produce an excess of mucus in the colon in certain patients. Just as certain stressful and emotional situations can make a person cry or perspire, so can these environmental stimuli cause excessive mucus in the stool. A car accident can produce mucus in one person and diarrhea in another.

QUESTION: How can you cure mucus colitis?

Mucus colitis can be cured by investigation into what food products cause an increased amount of mucus in the stool; or, a good history can reveal that the patient is under a stressful condition that is producing the excessive mucus. By elimination of the cause, plus some helpful medication, the excessive mucus production can be cleared up.

QUESTION: Should I worry if I pass visible mucus from my rectum?

ANSWER: Most of the time, passing an excessive amount of mucus which can easily be seen mixed in the stool does not alarm a physician unless there is blood mixed in the mucus. If a person passes a lot of mucus frequently he can lose some potassium and other elements, and this may harm the patient.

QUESTION: Do certain types of colonic tumors produce mucus in excess, so that one can see it?

ANSWER: Yes, the villous tumor of the colon and rectum produces mucus, but it rarely produces it in excess quantities so that it can be visualized; thus, a physician who obtains a history of a person passing excess mucus would think more of a dietary cause or psychosomatic cause before he would think of a tumor being the cause.

QUESTION: What are some of the more serious types of colitis?

ANSWER: Some of the more serious types of colitis are chronic ulcerative colitis and granulomatous colitis.

QUESTION: What is chronic ulcerative colitis?

ANSWER: This is a chronic disease of the colon that affects the lining of the colon and produces small ulcers that give the person the main symptom of bloody mucus.

QUESTION: What is the cause of chronic ulcerative colitis?

ANSWER: We have no known cause for chronic ulcerative colitis. We think that it possibly may be due to an abnormal antigen-antibody response in the body or possibly some abnormal bacteria or virus, but the cause at this time is unknown.

QUESTION: How does chronic ulcerative colitis affect the patient?

ANSWER: Patients usually start out in their teens or twenties by having several episodes of flu-like symptoms or upset stomach in one year. They go to one physician or various physicians who diagnose them as having the flu and treat them with common antibiotics. The various symptoms, such as diarrhea, bloody mucus, slight weight loss, nausea, and vomiting, continue until a physician examines the patient with a proctoscope and under direct vision—as well as by taking biopsies of the wall of the colon—diagnoses the patient to have chronic ulcerative disease.

QUESTION: What are the causes of spastic colitis and mucus colitis?

ANSWER: Spastic colitis can be brought on by tension and nerves, and if this is the true reason for spastic colitis, then it can be treated with psychotherapy and tranquilizers. Mucus colitis can be brought on also by tension and nerves, and possibly diet. This can also be treated by psychotherapy, diet, and possibly antibiotics.

QUESTION: What is the history of chronic ulcerative colitis in most patients?

ANSWER: This disease affects patients usually in their teens and twenties, and tends to have exacerbations that last several months and then remissions that last several months or several years.

QUESTION: When a patient with chronic ulcerative colitis has an attack, what are some of the symptoms?

ANSWER: Some of the symptoms are bloody mucus, multiple loose bowel movements, cramping abdominal pain, a feeling of fullness in the rectum, as though you were constipated, weight loss, and loss of appetite.

QUESTION: How are most of these patients treated?

ANSWER: Most people with chronic ulcerative colitis can be treated with medication and do very well. The medication consists of an intestinal antibiotic that is specific for this disease call Azulfidine. In conjunction with the Azulfidine, the patient can use either suppositories or small enemas with hydrocortisone in them or foams containing hydrocortisone injected into the rectum. Only as a last resort does the physician treat the patient with oral cortisone medication.

QUESTION: How is chronic ulcerative colitis diagnosed in a patient?

ANSWER: In cases of chronic ulcerative colitis, 95 percent of them will appear in the lower ten inches of the rectum; thus, a proctoscopic examination will usually identify or diagnose chronic ulcerative colitis; however, there may be skip areas in the colon when the rectum can look perfectly clear, and yet the disease can be three feet from the anal opening; thus, it would be helpful also to obtain a colonoscopy examination on these patients.

QUESTION: If the patient becomes very sick and does not respond to oral medication, diet, or even intravenous medication in the hospital, what is the next mode of treatment?

ANSWER: If the patient has irreversible changes in the colon lining and is not responding to medication and continues to get sicker, then this patient becomes an ideal candidate for surgery.

QUESTION: If chronic ulcerative colitis is to be treated by surgery, what is involved in this surgery?

ANSWER: There are two ways of treating the chronic ulcerative colitis in the colon and rectum. One is by removing the entire colon and rectum and performing an ileostomy.

An ileostomy, as discussed before, is a portion of small intestine that is brought out through the abdominal wall for approximately an inch, and the patient wears a bag for the rest of his life, because the patient evacuates constantly into this bag.

QUESTION: Are there other operations for this type of disease?

ANSWER: There are newer operations that are performed called "continent ileostomies," which are the so-called J-pouch or S-pouch type surgeries, and there are a lot of complications and a lot of morbidity with these operations.

QUESTION: If the patient is extremely sick and has his colon and rectum removed, does the patient automatically get well and become healthy and carry on a normal life?

ANSWER: Almost 100 percent of the people that have their colon and rectum removed will again function as a normal person with a small handicap called an ileostomy. They can carry on work at their place of employment, and they can also carry on normal sports activities within reason. They usually gain back their weight and in general have a normal lifestyle.

QUESTION: Do people with chronic ulcerative colitis have to be on the lookout for cancer of the colon more than the average person?

ANSWER: Yes. Those patients that have had chronic ulcerative colitis for as long as ten years or more have a 30 percent chance of getting a cancer of the colon and rectum over the average person who does not have chronic ulcerative colitis.

QUESTION: What happens if chronic ulcerative colitis is treated with medication and does not respond to this medication and the patient refuses surgery?

ANSWER: If the patient is on medication that is doing little good, and the patient refuses surgery, the ulcers in the lining of the colon can perforate and cause fistula formation, that is, sinus tracts between one piece of bowel and another piece of bowel, or this can cause abscess formation within the abdominal cavity, or this can cause intestinal obstruction and peritonitis, all of which are very serious and may lead to death.

QUESTION: What is the difference between chronic ulcreative colitis and the so-called "Crohn's disease" or "regional ileitis"?

ANSWER: Chronic ulcerative colitis is a disease we do not know the cause of, and it is generally confined to the colon and rectum. Crohn's disease or regional ileitis, which also we do not know the cause of, is usually confined to the terminal part of the small intestine called the "ileum," which is the portion of small intestine that goes into the right side of the colon. In Crohn's disease, the ileum is usually involved, along with a very small portion of the cecum or right colon.

QUESTION: What are the symptoms of Crohn's disease?

ANSWER: The symptoms and signs of Crohn's disease are usually pain and discomfort in the right lower quadrant of the abdomen, cramping abdominal pains, nausea and vomiting, chills and fever, and unexplained anal and rectal disease.

QUESTION: Can you explain the anorectal complications of Crohn's disease?

ANSWER: Yes. The anorectal complications of Crohn's disease usually consist of undulating fissures that are markedly infected and do not heal on their own, and which heal very slowly with surgery. There are fistulas that are not typical fistulas and in the female mostly involve the rectovaginal septum, producing a sinus tract between the rectum and vagina. These fistulas are almost impossible to heal with conservative treatment or with a diverting colostomy.

QUESTION: What is the treatment of choice for Crohn's disease, and in what age group does it usually occur?

ANSWER: Crohn's disease is usually seen in the teens and twenties of life, and the treatment of choice usually consists of medication including intestinal antibiotics, in addition to diet, and with cortisone only as a last resort.

QUESTION: If Crohn's disease does not respond to medical treatment, what is the alternative choice?

ANSWER: The alternative choice is to do surgery, which consists of either removing the affected part and joining the two good pieces of bowel together, such as the midportion of the ileum to the transverse colon; or, as a second choice in surgery, the affected part of the ileum can be bypassed by attaching the good part of the ileum to the transverse colon through an enterostomy, and this would bypass the affected part of the ileum, and the affected part would not have to be removed. This is usually done in very sick patients who cannot undergo lengthy operations.

QUESTION: Is it true that Crohn's disease can have skip areas in it?

ANSWER: Yes. A person whose small intestine is involved with Crohn's disease has the last eight to ten inches of the small intestine involved. This can be treated with medication or taken out by surgery, and the patient will recover; however, later on or at the same time the patient can have so-called skip areas. This means that one portion of the small intestine can be affected, then there can be a long normal piece of intestine, and then another five to six inches or five to six feet of intestine involved with the disease.

QUESTION: What is diverticular disease of the colon?

ANSWER: Approximately 20 percent of the people in the United States, which is about 45 million people, have so-called "pockets" that form out of the colonic wall called "diverticula." These small outpouchings, which are connected to the colon, can be completely asymptomatic throughout one's entire life.

QUESTION: Can these diverticular pockets become infected and become dangerous?

ANSWER: Yes. These colonic diverticula can become infected to the point where they may require surgery.

QUESTION: What causes diverticular disease?

ANSWER: We do not know why some people have diverticula and others do not; it is just a trait with some people.

QUESTION: Are there different types of diverticula in the colon?

ANSWER: Yes. The diverticula in the right side of the colon have wide necks entering into the pocket, and those on the left side of the colon have bottle-type necks entering into the diverticula. This is important because 99 percent of diverticulitis occurs on the left side of the colon.

QUESTION: Why do most of the infections in diverticular disease occur on the left side of the colon?

ANSWER: Since the diverticula have wide openings to them on the right side of the colon and since the waste material is liquid on the right side of the colon, the stool can flow in and out of these right-sided diverticula and they do not inspissate and become infected; however, as the stool goes around to the left side of the colon, it becomes a solid and it can be squeezed into the bottle-necked diverticula and cannot get out, and this may cause infection.

QUESTION: What part of the colon is the most common place for diverticula to become infected?

ANSWER: The most common place in the colon where diverticula get infected is called the "sigmoid colon," which is down in the left lower quadrant of your abdominal cavity.

QUESTION: In what age group is this disease most common?

ANSWER: This disease is most common in the age group of the sixties, seventies, and eighties, and rarely becomes a surgical disease and can mostly be treated with diet and antibiotics.

QUESTION: Can this disease occur in younger patients?

ANSWER: Yes. This disease can occur in the forties age group and the fifties age group, but when these patients have an attack, it is more serious, and the attacks may lead to an earlier surgery than if the patients were in an older age group.

QUESTION: How are most patients treated who have an attack of diverticulitis?

ANSWER: Most people who have a mild to moderate attack of diverticulitis are treated with oral antibiotics and a special low residue diet, and possibly a stool softener. Most of these patients will get over their attack at home within a week to ten days.

QUESTION: When should surgery be considered?

ANSWER: If a patient has multiple attacks in any one year's time and the home treatment of antibiotics and diet does not seem to be curing the patient as rapidly as it should, then it is time to discuss surgery with the patient.

QUESTION: In your practice, out of one hundred patients that you might see with diverticulitis, how many of them ever have to have surgery for this disease?

ANSWER: Less than five will ever have to have surgery for their disease. These are usually patients who are having several attacks a year that cause extreme left lower quadrant abdominal pain, chills and fever, and maybe some abdominal distention.

QUESTION: What kind of surgery does a patient have if he decides to have elective surgery to remove that portion of the colon that has diverticulitis?

ANSWER: The patient who wishes to have elective surgery on his colon for diverticulitis goes into the hospital and the colon is prepared with special antibiotics for approximately two days; then, the patient has major surgery, which requires the removal of approximately a foot to a foot and a half of colon that has the infected diverticulum in it. The two end pieces of colon are joined together, and after surgery the patient usually goes home within a week. The recovery time at home is about three more weeks, and then the patient may lead a normal life.

QUESTION: I have heard that sometimes temporary colostomies must be done in order to cure a patient of diverticulitis.

ANSWER: This is true. If the patient develops a ruptured diverticulum that causes an abscess around the colon, many times the infected piece of colon can be removed, but in order to protect the area that was joined together, a temporary colostomy must be done in order to detour the fecal stream away from the surgical resection.

QUESTION: How long does a patient usually have a temporary colostomy?

ANSWER: Most temporary colostomies are replaced back into the abdomen in two months. This requires about six to eight days in the hospital.

QUESTION: Is there much care to a temporary colostomy?

ANSWER: Actually, there is very little care to a temporary colostomy as opposed to a permanent colostomy. A temporary colostomy requires only a shower and then the application of a small plastic bag over the colostomy.

QUESTION: Can diverticulitis in a patient be a very serious disease?

ANSWER: Yes. Diverticulitis in a patient can be extremely serious, especially if the diverticulum has perforated. A perforated diverticulum may cause an abdominal abscess with either local or generalized peritonitis.

QUESTION: What food products should generally be avoided so that your diverticula do not become infected?

ANSWER: Most doctors feel that a low residue diet is the diet of choice when a person has diverticular disease, and certainly patients should not eat food products that contain husks, shells, seeds, or any fibrous material, which may inspissate into the bottle-necked diverticula and possibly abscess. Many patients have gotten the idea that because a high-fiber diet helps their elimination it must be good for certain diseases of the colon. This is myth when it comes to diverticulitis, especially as I have seen in my practice.

Chapter X

Transmitted Rectal Diseases

Section 1—Sexually Transmitted Rectal Diseases

QUESTION: What is the most common venereal disease seen and diagnosed in the anal canal?

ANSWER: Gonorrhea is the most prevalent venereal disease seen and diagnosed in the anal canal, and is the second most prevalent disease diagnosed in the human body after the common cold, which is number one.

QUESTION: How do you get gonorrhea in the rectum and anal canal?.

ANSWER: This is obtained by having anal intercourse with a person who is infected with gonorrhea.

QUESTION: How does a person know that they have gonorrhea of the rectum and anus?

ANSWER: The patient has such symptoms as bleeding from the rectum and passing a mucuslike discharge from the rectum. He also has a feeling of swelling down in the rectum. The patient may also have pain with a bowel movement.

QUESTION: What should you do if you have those symptoms of the rectum and anus, and how does the doctor diagnose the disease?

ANSWER: A person with those symptoms and signs should seek medical advice immediately. The doctor will examine the rectum and anus with an anoscope and a proctoscope, and he will obtain cultures of the walls of the rectum and anus. Also, on visualization of this area, the lining of the rectum and anus will be very red and will have mucus or pus clinging to the walls of the rectum and anus.

QUESTION: Is there a cure for gonorrhea of the rectum and anus?

ANSWER: Yes. At the time the doctor takes a culture of the rectum, he also obtains what we call a sensitivity test, which matches the bacteria to antibiotics, either oral or injectable, which best treat that particular bacteria, which in almost 95 percent of the cases will clear up the disease of gonorrhea of the rectum and anus.

QUESTION: What precautions should be taken in order not to get gonorrhea again in this manner?

ANSWER: If you are having anal intercourse with one partner, then he should definitely be checked for gonorrhea. A person should also avoid multiple sexual encounters with different partners. Also, a condom would be helpful.

QUESTION: Can one obtain gonorrhea from oral sex?

ANSWER: Yes, one can obtain gonorrhea from oral sex, and the patient will have a swollen lining of the mouth, including bleeding easily, and a mucous discharge from the lining of the mouth.

QUESTION: Is gonorrhea just as much a heterosexual disease as a homosexual disease?

ANSWER: Yes, gonorrhea is just as much a heterosexual disease as a homosexual disease.

QUESTION: Is syphilis still a prevalent disease in society?

ANSWER: Syphilis, although not publicized as much as it used to be, is still very prevalent in society and can be transmitted through heterosexual or homosexual intercourse.

QUESTION: What are the first outward signs of syphilis in the body?

ANSWER: Generally, one of the first signs of syphilis in the genital region can be a discharge either from the vaginal or rectal areas, and most common is a painless ulceration in the vicinity of the vagina, rectum, or penile area; this ulceration is called a chancre. Other symptoms can be chills and fever, as well as rash.

QUESTION: Is there a cure for syphilis?

ANSWER: Yes. Large doses of antibiotics (especially penicillin) can cure this disease.

QUESTION: Are warts around the anal and perianal area and in the anal canal a venereal disease?

ANSWER: There is one type of wart around the anal and perianal area and in the anal canal that is called "condyloma latum." This is definitely a venereal wart and is usually treated by excision of the wart and antibiotics. There is a more common wart around the anal and perianal area that I see every day in my office called "condyloma acuminatum." This is a venereal wart only if it is obtained by anal intercourse. This can also be treated by excising the wart and burning the base.

QUESTION: Why is this condyloma acuminatum not considered a venereal wart?

ANSWER: This type of wart is the same wart that people get on their fingers if they keep their hands in water a lot or, also, it is the same type of wart that is in the female vagina or any place on the body that stays warm and moist. This type of wart is considered a venereal wart if obtained by sexual contact.

QUESTION: How can you tell definitely if a condyloma acuminatum was obtained by anal intercourse?

ANSWER: You can tell that these warts were obtained by anal intercourse if the warts are in the anal canal. If the warts are in the anal canal, it is diagnostic that this is how this patient acquired the warts. If the warts are not in the anal canal and are merely in the perianal area, then this patient may not have had anal intercourse.

QUESTION: Are warts in a female's vagina considered venereal?

ANSWER: Warts in a woman's vagina are rarely considered venereal warts because they are very common in this area; however, they may have obtained them from intercourse with a partner who has warts.

QUESTION: Can a person get warts from a toilet seat or a dirty towel in a gymnasium or by taking a whirlpool bath with other people?

ANSWER: No, a person may not pick up the disease in this manner, because the virus, unless it starts to grow, will last for only a few seconds on material such as described; however, a person may pick up warts in such places that give a colonic lavage, using the same enema tip on one person after another, without proper cleansing.

QUESTION: Is surgery the only way to get rid of anal warts?

ANSWER: No. A doctor might place a special solution on these warts that may either completely get rid of them or control them. This is usually done in the office with very little pain and is usually done where there are only a few warts and they are not in the anal canal.

QUESTION: How effective is treating the warts in the office with, say, a substance such as podophyllum?

ANSWER: If the warts are no bigger than two millimeters in size and they are just confined to the anal and perianal area and are not in the anal canal, then this treatment is fairly reliable, but on many occasions the patient must come back to the office for many visits for constant application of the medication.

QUESTION: If surgery is the treatment of choice in larger and more numerous warts, what is the recurrence rate of these warts?

ANSWER: The recurrence rate of anal warts depends on many factors. One of the factors is if the patient continues to have further contact with another person who has warts. Another factor is that at the time of surgery there may be warts that are microscopic and cannot be seen grossly with the naked eye and of course are not removed at that time. Another factor is that some warts may be so small that they are missed and not removed at the time of surgery and will continue to grow in the postoperative period. This surgery is done on an outpatient basis, under anesthesia, and takes only a few minutes. Usually the patient can go home within two hours from start to finish.

QUESTION: What is the best way for the physician and patient to handle the postoperative period so that the warts are gone forever?

ANSWER: Two main factors will help in getting rid of the warts and keeping them gone forever. One is for the patient not to have any more anal and rectal intercourse. The other factor is for the physician to follow the patient postoperatively in the office for at least six months, checking the patient both in the anal and perianal area and in the anal canal. If the doctor finds a wart two or three months postoperatively, he can easily remove that wart in the office.

QUESTION: Are warts contagious?

ANSWER: Yes, warts are contagious and can be passed from one person to another very readily.

QUESTION: Is there a vaccine that one can take that will ensure that a person will not get any more warts?

ANSWER: There have been some research studies in the past involving a person donating the warts that have been excised from him. A vaccine is made out of these warts, and the patient is immunized with this vaccine made from his own warts; however, several years of study with this vaccine have not proven fruitful.

QUESTION: Do the anal warts that are medically called condylomata acuminata ever turn into a malignancy?

ANSWER: In my practice I have never seen any of these warts become malignant, but in the literature I have come across one article in the past twenty-four years where a doctor had one patient in whom, supposedly, a portion of the warts turned into a malignancy.

QUESTION: If a few of the cases that you see in your office over the years are not transmitted sexually, then how does the patient acquire these warts?

ANSWER: These warts that we have been talking about commonly occur in areas on the body that are moist and warm, such as under the breasts of women whose breasts are large and pendulous. Also, in fat people who have large, fatty abdominal aprons, condyloma warts will occur under these aprons in the groin area. Too, warts can occur in the axillary areas on some fat people. If a patient has a draining anal abscess or an open anal fissure that keeps the anal and perianal area moist with either serum or pus, this also can contribute to a perfect environment for growing warts.

Section 2—AIDS

QUESTION: What is AIDS?

ANSWER: AIDS stands for "acquired immune deficiency syndrome," which means that the defense mechanisms of the body have been broken down by a foreign virus.

QUESTION: How does a person get AIDS?

ANSWER: AIDS is predominantly a sexually transmitted disease and can be obtained most commonly by anal and rectal intercourse.

QUESTION: How else can somebody obtain AIDS?

ANSWER: AIDS can also be obtained by blood transfusions, by using needles that have not been sterilized, by salvia, and by vaginal intercourse.

QUESTION: Approximately how many people have AIDS in the United States, and is it a fatal disease?

ANSWER: As this book is written, approximately thirty-five thousand people have been reported to have AIDS and approximately twenty thousand people have died from AIDS. AIDS is definitely 100 percent fatal.

QUESTION: Are the people in the United States concerned about AIDS and its treatment?

ANSWER: Yes. AIDS is the number one health concern in the United States and possibly around the world. More and more money is being allocated by the various governments in the world for scientific research to find out how to cure this 100 percent fatal disease.

QUESTION: What are scientists finding so complex about the incubation period of this disease?

ANSWER: The complexity of the incubation of this disease is the fact a person can have been infected years ago with the AIDS virus and yet not break out with the actual infection for years to come.

QUESTION: How does a person who has no idea he has AIDS become aware that he might have this virus?

ANSWER: The most likely situation is for a person who has been infected with the AIDS virus, yet is asymptomatic, to get a common infection such as a cold. The AIDS virus then attacks the defensive mechanism of the person's body, and the body has tremendous trouble getting rid of its infection because its defense mechanism has been broken down by the AIDS virus; thus, such things as kidney infections, pneumonia, and even the common cold can become extremely serious in a person with AIDS.

QUESTION: After a person feels that he has come in contact with a person with AIDS or had a sexual encounter with a person with AIDS, how long does it take for the AIDS antibody test to prove positive?

ANSWER: The incubation period for the AIDS virus is approximately six weeks to three months, and at this time the AIDS anitbodies can be detected on testing.

QUESTION: So far, is there any cure for AIDS?

ANSWER: No, there is no cure for AIDS, but there is a drug on the market called AZT, which may prolong the life of an AIDS patient; however, this drug can be very expensive, as much as ten thousand dollars a year, for its administration.

QUESTION: What is the mechanism of the AZT medication in an AIDS patient?

ANSWER: The AZT treatment inhibits AIDS virus cells from multiplying; however, it does have side effects. It is toxic to the bone marrow and tends in some people to damage the bone marrow. It will prolong the life of some patients but will not cure them. As mentioned above, this treatment is very expensive.

QUESTION: How can a person keep from getting AIDS?

ANSWER: The number one prevention in order not to get AIDS is to abstain from all sexual activity. The second best way of not obtaining AIDS is the use of a condom. There are two types of condoms that are advertised in the stores. One is the natural type condom, which is very dangerous because it is slightly porous and will allow the virus and semen to penetrate through the condom. The other condom is the latex condom, and only if this condom is torn is it dangerous.

QUESTION: What is one of the worst things that a person can do to contract the AIDS virus?

ANSWER: One of the worst things a person can do is to have multiple indiscriminate sex partners without the use of a condom.

QUESTION: Can this disease be spread by merely shaking hands or drinking at the fountains after an AIDS patient?

ANSWER: No, it is felt that the spread of AIDS is not a casual situation and that hugging a person or shaking hands with a person infected with AIDS will not transmit the virus.

QUESTION: What are some of the things that I can do to lower my risk of getting AIDS?

ANSWER: (1) Abstain from sex completely. (2) Do not have sex with people known to have AIDS. (3) Do not have sex with people who are positive for the AIDS test or suspected of having AIDS. (4) Do not have sex with partners you do not know very well. (5) Avoid using injections and various instruments immediately following a drug user's having used the same instruments. (6) Use a condom at all times while having rectal or vaginal sex.